Gu

An Ancient Chinese Technique for Facial and Skin Self Healing

Marvin Valerie Georgia

Healing Energy 4 ALL
(403) 308-2041
cindy@healingenergy4all.ca

ISBN: 978-1-63750-333-1

Free Bonus

Download **"The Magic Of Starting Over"** Ebook For **FREE!**

Did you know that the greatest barrier to success is the fear of failure? Fear of failure stops people from taking risks that might lead to success and triumph in overcoming obstacles.

Fear is part of human nature…

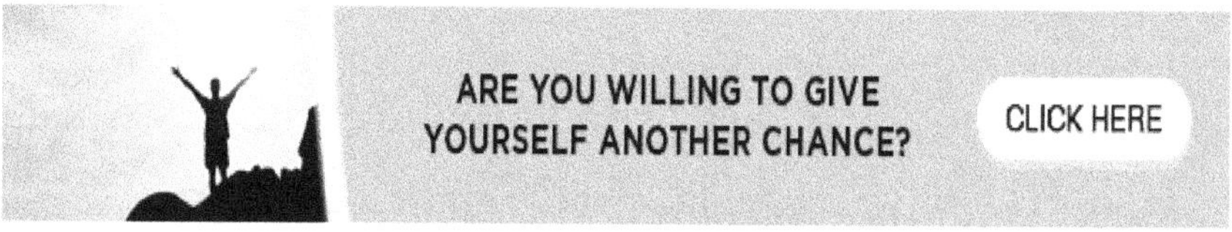

Click the image above to **Download the Book**, and also Subscribe for Free books, giveaways, and new releases by me. https://mayobook.com/marvin

My Other Books

I recommend these books to you, they will be of help, check them out after reading this book.

1. **Acupuncture:** A Practical Guide to Enjoying a Perfect Health with Natural Medicine
2. **Alcohol Control:** The Guide to Overcoming Alcoholism, and Breaking Free From Alcohol Addiction (Alcoholism Recovery)
3. **Alcohol Detox:** The Guide to Safely Clean Up Your Lifestyle, Detoxify & Maintain Healthy Body Without Drugs (Alcoholism Recovery)
4. **Anger Management:** The Inside Out Parent Child Interaction Therapy (PCIT) Approach to Managing Anger Issues and Emotions (Anger Management Program Book 1)
5. **CBT - Cognitive Behavioral Therapy:** The Clinician & Parental Guide to Managing Anger, Anxiety, ADHD, Trauma, Conduct Disorder, and Overcoming Negative
6. **ADHD:** A Practical Parental & Educator Multimodal Guide to Helping Children with ADHD Break Through Barriers and Develop Ability to Regulate their Behaviors and Strengths
7. **Asthma Relief:** How To Relieve Your Asthma Symptoms And Live The Life You Deserve with Natural Remedies
8. **7-Day Cleanse and Detox:** The Ultimate Guide To Getting Clean And Feeling Good!

9. **Cognitive Behavioral Therapy for Conduct Disorders and Personality Disorders:** How to Use CBT to Help Kids with Emotional Disorders
10. **Dyslexia:** Things You Don't Know About Dyslexia Learning Difficulties (But Should)
11. **Fear:** Overcoming and Facing Your Fear & Succeeding at Anything
12. **Sensory Processing Disorder:** How to Help Kids Cope with Sensory Issues (SPD)
13. **How to Parent - Toddler Discipline:** Raising Happy, Well-Behaved Kids by Taming the Tantrum Monster
14. **Childhood Trauma Healing:** Understanding & Healing Traumatic Experiences that Affect Children's Wellbeing (Emotional Trauma and Recovery Guide)
15. **Gua Sha:** An Ancient Chinese Technique for Facial and Skin Self Healing
16. **Potty Chair for Boys and Girls:** Potty Training in One Week, and The Ultimate Potty Buying Guide
17. **ADHD in Kids: ADHD in Kids:** What Parents and Teachers Should Know About Attention Deficit Hyperactivity Disorder

Table of Contents

Introduction

The Gua Sha technique was originally developed as a way to stimulate internal energy circulation, which can help ease symptoms of arthritis and rheumatism, as well as enhance healing of the body.

By applying pressure on the skin using a special technique called Gua Sha, a person can release toxins from the body as well as remove impurities and stimulate blood flow and lymphatic circulation.

Traditional Chinese medicine holds that if we are stressed and anxious our skin cannot heal well. We must become calm to help our skin heal. This ancient technique uses pressure and heat to open blocked energy channels. It is used to treat chronic acne, pimples and wrinkles, and also improve the overall health of the skin.

A popular form of alternative medicine, gua sha is an ancient technique developed in China. This self-care practice has been practiced for thousands of years to help improve blood flow, increase the energy flow throughout the body and treat muscle spasms.

"Gua sha" is an ancient Chinese technique for facial and

skin self healing. It has been used by the Chinese for hundreds of years.

Today, it's being taught to Westerners as a way to promote health and rejuvenation of the skin and body. There are several reasons why gua sha is effective, including its ability to draw out impurities and toxins, to stimulate the lymphatic system, and to stimulate blood circulation.

The Gua Sha technique is based on the belief that there are two *'energy meridians'* or channels through which healing energy travels through the body.

There are five channels, one for each of the five elements, and each channel is connected to a specific part of the body.

The first channel is the ***Governing Channel***, which runs from the top of the head down the spine and connects to the bladder, liver, gall bladder and stomach.

The second is the ***Middle Channel***, which starts at the center of the chest and moves down the front of the body to the navel and the spleen.

The third channel is the ***Conception Vessel***, which starts in the area of the heart and connects to the lungs, the kidneys and the bladder.

The fourth channel is the ***Pericardium Vessel***, which starts at the back of the heart and runs to the palms of the hands and feet.

The fifth channel is the ***Renal Vessel***, which starts in the kidney area and travels down the thighs and legs to the tip of the toes.

Gua sha is an ancient Chinese technique used to massage or knead certain points on the body that correspond to specific organs. It is said to reduce pain and improve function. It is believed to increase **chi** (or life force), blood circulation, and lymphatic drainage.

Gua sha techniques include both *soft and hard strokes*. Hard strokes work to break up tissue and relieve congestion. Soft strokes are used to stimulate the skin and to encourage the flow of **qi**, or life energy. Gua sha can be done either internally or externally, and can be done with the hands, fingers, palms, or a device called a ***ball***. The ball is a small object usually made from metal or plastic that has small indentations or cavities on its surface. The purpose of a gua sha ball is to assist in stimulating the skin and helping the user perform the techniques properly.

A component of Traditional Chinese Medicine, ***Gua-sha*** (TCM), *"Scraping," "spooning," and "coining"* are other terms for this practice. It is employed in the medical field as a tool for removing dead skin cells from the surface of the skin. ***Tribo-effleurage*** is the French term for the method of administering this drug. Using a massage instrument to scrape the top layer of your skin, gua-sha is an all-natural alternative therapy that works to increase blood flow. Using this traditional Chinese therapeutic approach, you may improve your overall health and also address concerns like chronic pain.

An expert doing the Gua-sha technique applies massage essential oil to your skin before using a smooth-edged tool known as a *Gua-therapeutic massage tool*, to scrape your skin layer in a downward motion frequently in order to stimulate the microcirculation of the smooth cells, which increases blood flow. Gua-sha ought to handle stagnant energy called ***chi.*** This "***chi***" is thought to be responsible for swellings in any portion of the body, and Gua-sha can be used to deal with it. Many illnesses associated with persistent pain are caused by swelling. Massage on the skin's surface is thought to assist in dispersing this energy, alleviate discomfort, and speed healing.

On the back, buttocks, neck, hands, and legs, gua-sha is typically conducted. Even as a cosmetic procedure, a modest variant of it is administered to the facial skin. It is possible that your specialist will begin with gentle pressure and gradually increase the strength to determine how much pressure your body can withstand.

As you read further, learn how to effectively apply gua sha, a centuries old technique from China, to naturally remove acne, reduce scarring, heal scars, treat rosacea, clear pores, improve skin tone, and even reduce wrinkles.

Chapter 1

What is Face Gua Sha?

Face Traditional Chinese Medicine uses Gua-Sha, a scraping massage technique. It began as a self-administered treatment to improve blood circulation, lymphatic stagnation, and alleviate muscle tension. An easier to use variant was eventually developed for facial skin, using a gentle glide to lift and smooth the skin's surface. With light upward and downward pressure, tools of various forms made of crystal *(such as jade or rose quartz)* can be found mixed together on the ground.

The goal is to promote lymphatic drainage into the neck and deliver new blood and nutrients to the skin's surface for a healthy glow while also de-plumping the facial skin. Your skin's microcirculation is enhanced when you gently scrape your skin layer, which helps to eliminate congestion, stimulate cell regeneration, and brighten your complexion. If you have acne or want to remove acne scars, this flurry of blood offers nutrients that promote cell regeneration and tissue healing, making it considerably more effective.

A 5-minute addition to your morning or nighttime skin care routine that will lift and shine your face every time is an incredible value.

Benefit of Gua-sha

Using Gua-sha Cosmetics has many advantages. Acne and irritated skin can both be exacerbated by a lymphatic liquid called gua-sha, which builds up under the skin of the face and is responsible for removing toxins.

Gua-Sha performs the following actions:

- Reduces the appearance of drooping skin by concealing the muscles beneath the skin's surface.
- It firms and moisturizes the top layer of your skin.
- Reduces overall stress by relieving muscle tension in the face (the body enters a parasympathetic state, which is ideal for those who have trouble falling asleep).
- Blood circulation and flow are improved.
- Dark circles and under-eye bags are caused in part by sluggish blood flow.

- Acne scars and blemishes can be reduced by using this product.
- To prevent and remove existing wrinkles, as well as assist in preventing new wrinkles from forming,
- It also reduces the appearance of facial puffiness.
- In a matter of seconds, it works to lift and plump your skin.
- Because of this, post-treatment serums can go deeper into the skin than usual.
- Tight muscles or fascia might induce a sore throat and headache.

How to Practice Gua Sha at Home

Starting with the throat/jaw and working your way up implies that you begin lymphatic drainage at the least expensive level, so that when you reach your forehead and vision area, the liquid and poisons have a funnel to drain into.

Even while the lymphatic system is important, if your skin gets excessively red, it's time for some company rather than focusing on the lymphatic system. Due to the proximity of your lymphatic vessels to the top of your body, your tools should be slanted at approximately 15-20 degrees, virtually smooth on your skin, so that you don't stab yourself and enjoy the soft pull that plays a component in the lifting action.

When cleaning your neck, be sure to scrape the outer edges of your facial skin and sweep downward from the guts so that lymph fluid flows properly into the nodes above your collarbone.

How Important is Your Lymphatic System?

Your lymphatic system is just as important as your circulatory system, if not more so. Unlike the circulatory system, the lymphatic system does not have a built-in pump to pump and clear the blood. Exercise, massage therapy, and a healthy diet all help to maintain lymph flow, so it's simple to benefit from this modern way of life.

TCM and Ayurveda, two ancient systems of medicine, believe stasis in the lymphatic system to be the first place to look when someone is ill. Western medicine has only recently begun to completely understand the lymphatic system. Other countries, such as Germany, use specific lymphatic drainage techniques to treat a variety of ailments, including fibrocystic breast disease, allergies, persistent sinusitis, arthritis, eczema, heart disease, and more. The *American Medical Association (AMA)* has traditionally ignored lymphatic stagnation as a cause of disease.

In order to tell if your lymphatic system is sluggish, you can think of your blood as the tap, and your lymph as the drain. The fact that your blood is constantly pumping means that your valves are always in use. However, they sprint right into the area where it's still not certain that it will. There are lymphatic vessels that receive waste products from the bloodstream that are too big to be eliminated by the organs of the liver, kidneys, or skin. As a result, stagnation and sickness arise when these "drains" aren't moving.

Poor lymphatic circulation can be caused by a variety of factors, including:

- **Stress**: It's important to note that the chemistry of stress is degenerative and lymphocongested.

Working too many hours without taking enough time off might harm your lymphatic system, digestion, and liver Qi.

- **Imbalances in the Digestive System**: Because of the "Gut Associated Lymph Tissue" that surrounds the digestive tract, irritation of the intestinal villi, attributed to inflammatory foods and poor digestion, causes congestion in the lymphatic system (GALT). Check out the rest of this book for 11 unusual (but simple) ways to improve your digestion. I've outlined the four most common causes of bad digestion and the remedies for each of them so that you can get more in-depth answers.
- **Deficiencies:** The lymphatic system is affected by nutrient deficits, particularly those involving iodine. If you live in a pesticide-sprayed society, you need iodine to keep your lymph nodes healthy and mobile. See my post on the health benefits of seaweed.
- **Emotions/Religion:** Shame, a lack of enjoyment in life, despair, and other repressed feelings are all symptoms of a dysfunctional emotional or

religious system.

- **Inactivity:** Because this lymph doesn't have a pump, it relies on you to keep it moving. Inactivity and sitting at a desk all day are bad for your lymphatic system.
- **Diet:** Eat right or avoid the lymph blitz with the right food choices. The lymph is negatively affected by processed sugars (corn syrup) and white flour.

The Face Gua-Sha is One little piece of the lymphatic puzzle, but it helps get things going if you have persistent sinus mucus buildup concerns.

The following are some suggestions for increasing lymphatic circulation:

- Take daily walks, especially after meals (even if it's only for ten minutes).
- Eat the oranges' white parts! (Click that to know more about my post on this).
- Eat meals with a reddish hue (pure cranberry juice, blueberries, and raspberries).
- Reduce the number of times per day that you'sit

back'. For just a few minutes a day, brush your teeth using a dry brush.

Chapter 2

Beauty Restored - The Advantages of Face Gua Sha

Make a dramatic change to your complexion with face massage therapy. You can learn a lot about someone just by looking at their face, not just by seeing how they're pulling or how they're reacting to the sensation right away. According to Chinese medicine, your attractiveness is an external representation of your interior health, and therefore, your health and fitness will be inscribed on your face.

Your general health will definitely improve as a result of our beauty regimens. A lot of long-standing Chinese wisdom has been condensed into a few potent one-minute practices by our founder and resident physician, Katie. They may be fast and convenient, and they may be easily integrated into our modern lifestyles, allowing us to transform our health and exercise routines into a healthy, glowing, and radiant tone.

Recreating Your Optimal Appearance

We're going to present three well-known Chinese methods for enhancing your physical appearance, and because we've already processed them, they should only take a few minutes to complete. It's one minute for each of us.

They are *Àn-fa (press-hold), gua-sha(press stroke), and acupressure (press-turn).*

It has been used for a long time in Chinese face massage therapy, and it is known for its calming and healing properties.

According to our research, 82% of women noticed a difference after just one minute of use.

Àn-fa

In this procedure, pressing and supporting the jade Beauty RestorerTM over your face may help reduce swelling and improve lymphatic drainage.

If you have tired eyes, puffy eyes, or twitching eye muscles, use the sweetness restorerTM on the area around your eyes to alleviate these symptoms. Stress-related symptoms such as headaches, flushes, skin conditions, and pounding temples can be relieved by using the jade tool on the affected area.

Gua-Sha

A simple press and heart stroke along the contours of your face, as illustrated in the video, is Gua-Sha. For decades, Asian women have relied on this beauty procedure. It's known for its ability to boost blood flow beneath the skin's surface, bringing in nourishment and boosting collagen production.

For example, instead of applying an anti-aging cream or serum, you're engaging your body to nourish your skin layer from the inside out. Studies have shown that this self-massage technique increases circulation by 100%.

Collagen production is stimulated, muscles are relaxed, and blood and lymphatic flow are dramatically increased by this treatment. You'll notice an overall improvement in your skin's tone and appearance.

Acupressure

A great way to help your internal organs is to use acupressure on your face. According to Chinese medicine, the appearance of your organs is a reflection of your total health, not the other way around.

Chapter 3

Gua Sha Tools & How to Use Them

Gua-Sha scrapers were once made of bones and even cow horns in the past. One day, someone told me that cow horns are wonderful carriers of vigor. I don't know if the myth is genuine, but I'd like to believe that telepathic cows exist. The fact that crystals are still used today is a good thing because they are said to emit energy as well.

The following is a list of the top resources to keep in mind:

1. Bian Stone

According to traditional Chinese medicine, Bian stones are the most effective tools for Gua-sha therapy due to their high number of ultrasonic pulsations as well as their ability to gather the highest frequencies. The five basic medical methods of the "Yellow Emperor," a deity in Chinese religious beliefs, are listed in the "Nei Jing," a historical Chinese medical magazine. "Acupuncture, moxibustion, natural medication, Qigong, and Bian rock therapy." It's amazing to think that Bian Rock Treatment existed before acupuncture, but it does.

Authentic Gua-Sha requires the usage of Bian rocks.

2. Jade

In terms of Gua-sha gadgets, jade comes in a close second. It is said to have qi energy that is almost as strong as your own. As a result, it's perfect for use in therapeutic procedures. Traditional Gua-sha tools were unavailable to barefoot doctors in China in the early days, so they used remnants from jade carvers to make their own tools. The medicinal properties of jade are still well known today.

3. Buffalo Horn

Sibin, China, is the only place to find authentic Bian rocks. Buffalo horn is a fantastic alternative if you can't get Bian rocks.

A buffalo horn's acrid/salty flavor and chilly properties are used in Chinese medicine. Acridity improves qi and blood circulation, provides nourishment, and lubricates. The salinity relaxes, loosens, and softens stiffness in a variety of ways. Warmth is dissipated and toxins are expelled by exposure to cold temperatures.

If you're concerned about where they're sourced from, jade, natural stone, and steel are all alternatives to buffalo horns.

4. Stainless Steel

Device Assisted Soft Cell Mobilization (DASCM) is a popular choice for medical-grade stainless tools, which are just a modern development of Gua-Sha. To get the most up-to-date tools, look into stainless steel and titanium implements.

5. Rose Quartz

Open the gut chakra with rose quartz, and you'll feel better. It's a delightful stone in the form of a delicate red coloration.

It's smooth and heavy, just like a Gua-Sha tool would be. The buffalo horn, or bian rock, on the other hand, is said to be difficult to handle and pick up by some. Gua-Sha can be performed with any object, be it a coin, a spoon, or a cover. Having the greatest materials and skills makes the entire experience easier and more memorable, as you use tools that become a part of your personal history.

Stress and disease management will be more natural, like how people have recovered in the past, rather than relying on drugs or other vices that only work for a short time.

Gua-Sha Jade Stone

The Eastern Botox, or Eastern Facelift, for the face and neck is called Gua-Sha for the grounds. When applied to the face, this traditional Chinese medicine treatment has the following effects:

- It firms up your drooping facial muscles.
- It reduces the appearance of wrinkles and fine lines on your face.
- Age spots and other skin discolorations are lightened, and your skin tone becomes rosier and more radiant.
- Moreover, it aids in the removal of acne, rosacea, and other skin illnesses on your face.

Konjac Face Sponge - Pure

A 100% pure konjac sponge deep cleans, removes blackheads, and gently exfoliates your skin. It is ideal for all skin types. Because of their initial web-like structure, vegetable fibers are able to stimulate blood flow and promote the renewal of skin cells.

How to use:

Before using, thoroughly clean the sponge.As a general rule, we recommend submerging it in water and squeezing it regularly. It's best to let the sponge soak up as much water as possible before using it on your face or body.

Exfoliate dead skin cells and deep-cleanse your face and body by gently massaging in a circular motion. Exhausted skin will be re-energized and renewed by the massage. If desired, you can add soap or cleaning solution to the sponge, although this step is not required.

If your sponge looks worn out or starts to break down after a year, replace it. Please have it changed. The sponge will survive longer if it is given proper care.

Konjac Face Sponge - Bamboo Charcoal

The Konjac Sponge with Bamboo Charcoal is enriched with activated carbon, which thoroughly cleans pores to remove blackheads and dirt and grime while absorbing excess oils and toxins. Acne-causing bacteria are killed by this natural antioxidant, which is also an effective treatment for the condition.

How to use:

The sponge should be well cleaned before use. As a general rule, we recommend submerging it in water and squeezing it regularly. Before applying it to your skin, wet the sponge if it is completely dry.

Exfoliate dead skin cells and deep-cleanse your face and body by gently massaging in a circular motion. Exhausted skin will be re-energized and renewed by the massage. If desired, a bar of soap or cleansing solution can be inserted inside the sponge.

If your sponge looks worn out or starts to break down

after a year, replace it. Please have it changed. The sponge will survive longer if it is given proper care.

Konjac Face Sponge - Green Tea Herb

To protect your skin from the destructive effects of free radicals, green tea extract is naturally rich in antioxidants that have a cell-protecting action. If you want to keep your skin from aging, you can use this natural ingredient to soften and plump it up, making it ideal for those who want to maintain their youthful appearance.

How to use:

The sponge should be well cleaned before use. As a general rule, we recommend submerging it in water and squeezing it regularly. It's best to let the sponge soak up as much water as possible before using it on your face or body.

Exfoliate dead skin cells and deep-cleanse your face and body by gently massaging in a circular motion. Exhausted skin will be re-energized and renewed by the massage. If desired, you can add soap or cleaning solution to the sponge, although this step is not required.

If your sponge looks worn out or starts to break down after a year, replace it. Please have it changed. The sponge will survive longer if it is given proper care.

Konjac Face Sponge - Folks from France Pink Clay

It's the perfect Konjac sponge to use when you're exposed to the extremes of air conditioning, direct sunlight, and central heating. It cleanses even the most fragile skin and has a softening and plumping effect on your skin's appearance by improving elasticity.

How to use:

Before using, thoroughly clean the sponge.As a general rule, we recommend submerging it in water and squeezing it regularly. It's best to let the sponge soak up as much water as possible before using it on your face or body.

Exfoliate dead skin cells and deep-cleanse your face and body by gently massaging in a circular motion.

Exhausted skin will be re-energized and renewed by the massage. If desired, you can add soap or cleaning solution to the sponge, although this step is not required.

If your sponge looks worn out or starts to break down after a year, replace it. Please have it changed. The sponge will survive longer if it is given proper care.

Konjac Face Sponge - Lavender

Using a lavender-infused Konjac Face Sponge can help with relaxation and detoxification while also aiding in the body's ability to heal. To soothe the skin, this gorgeous blossom has a powerful ability to relax and relieve stress and worry.

How to use:

Before using, thoroughly clean the sponge.As a general rule, we recommend submerging it in water and squeezing it regularly. It's best to let the sponge soak up as much water as possible before using it on your face or body.

Exfoliate dead skin cells and deep-cleanse your face and

body by gently massaging in a circular motion. Exhausted skin will be re-energized and renewed by the massage. If desired, you can add soap or cleaning solution to the sponge, although this step is not required.

If your sponge looks worn out or starts to break down after a year, replace it. Please have it changed. The sponge will survive longer if it is given proper care.

Chapter 4

Advantages of Gua Sha

For chronic pain conditions, including arthritis and fibromyalgia, gua-sha is typically used to reduce swelling. It is also utilized for muscular and joint discomfort.

A variety of conditions, such as the following, may benefit from the use of gua-sha.

1. HBV (Hepatitis B)

Hepatitis B is a virus infection that causes inflammation of the liver, liver damage, and scarring of the liver. According to studies, gua-sha has been shown to alleviate chronic liver inflammation.

Liver enzymes, which indicate inflammation in the liver, were monitored in a well-respected study. He was given Gua-sha medicine and saw a decrease in his liver enzymes after just 48 hours of treatment. Some specialists, on the other hand, believe that Gua-sha can help reduce liver edema and, as a result, the risk of liver damage. There is still more to be done.

2. Headaches caused by migraines

Even after you've tried many "over-the-counter drugs," Gua-sha may help alleviate your migraines. According to a credible source, a 72-year-old woman with persistent migraines was relieved of her symptoms after only two weeks of receiving Gua-sha treatment, indicating that this age-old treatment method could be an effective solution.

3. Engorgement of the breasts

Breast engorgement, or overfilling of the chest with milk, is a common condition for many breastfeeding mothers. This typically starts in the first few weeks of breastfeeding. Inflammation and soreness in the mother's breast make it harder for the baby to latch. However, this is a temporary state of affairs.

A study claims that Gua-sha is given to pregnant women from the first day they are admitted to a healthcare institution until they are discharged. Breastfeeding became easier for women who took gua-sha medicine in the weeks after they gave birth because they no longer had to deal with engorgement, or breast fullness and pain.

4. Pain in the neck

For chronic throat pain, the Gua-sha method is an excellent remedy. In order to evaluate the effectiveness of the therapy, 48 individuals were divided into two groups. To ease the pain in their throats, one group received gua-sha treatment, while the other employed a thermal heat pad. There was a significant difference in the level of pain reported by the two groups after one week of treatment.

5. Tourette's syndrome

Involuntary movements, such as tics on the face and neck, and verbal outbursts are all signs of Tourette's syndrome. People with Tourette's syndrome may benefit from a combination of gua-sha and other treatments.

He suffered from Tourette's syndrome at the age of 9 and had acupuncture, gua-sha, and other natural herbs, and his symptoms were reduced by 70 percent. Though he was found to be positive, more research is needed.

6. The Premenopausal syndrome:

Pre-menopausal affects women nearing menopause.

The following are some of the symptoms:

- Sleep disorder
- Periods that are not regular
- Anxiety
- Fatigue
- Feelings of ecstasy

In some women with premenopausal symptoms, gua-sha has been demonstrated to be beneficial. The study included 80 premenopausal women. For eight weeks, patients in the procedure group received normal therapy along with 15 gua-sha treatments. *Those in the control group received no additional treatment.*

As compared to the control group, the participants in the study who were actively involved reported fewer symptoms like insomnia, anxiety, weariness, headaches, and hot flashes at the study's end.

According to experts, gua-sha therapy may be deemed

safe and beneficial for certain symptoms.

Does Gua Sha have any Side effects?

Gua-sha is safe because it is an all-natural therapeutic remedy. Because the process involves massaging or scraping your skin with a massage therapy tool and breaking tiny arteries known as capillaries on the surface of your skin, it may cause some bruising and some blood loss on your skin, but it is not believed to be painful. Most bruises fade away within a few days.

Short-term indentation of the skin is a common side effect of gua-sha treatments.

Adopt these three measures in order to protect yourself:

- Because gua-sha therapy could spread blood-borne infections if there is bleeding, technicians need to clean their tools between patients to keep them safe.
- Be cautious if you've had surgery within the previous six weeks.
- People who have problems with their blood clotting or who are taking blood thinners should not try to get gua-sha.

Chapter 5

Uses of Gua-sha

The following are several methods for gua-sha meditation:

- To alleviate muscle and joint discomfort, gua-sha is commonly used in Chinese medicine. These are called musculoskeletal disorders, and they include things like back pain, tendon stress, and carpal tunnel symptoms.
- As practitioners claim, gua-sha also aids in reducing inflammation, preventing disease, and improving skin tone and texture. Gua-sha can be used to treat a cold, a fever, or a lung condition.
- Injuries to the body, such as gua-sha bruises, are referred to as "micro-trauma," and this term is used frequently. These elicit an immune response, which may aid in the separation of scar tissue. Fibrosis, which happens when your body builds up too much connective tissue as it heals, can also be helped by small injuries.
- When connective cells are unable to move bones,

physiotherapists may utilize IASTM. This may be due to repetitive stress damage or another issue. There are other therapies like stretching and conditioning exercises that can be used in conjunction with gua-sha.

Great Things about Gua Sha

Gua-sha is being tested on a new group of people to see if it has any effect. They include:

- Women nearing menopause.
- Those who suffer from computer-related neck aches may benefit from using a guitar's neck.
- For men who lift weights, to aid in recovery after exercise.
- Women experiencing premenopausal symptoms such as excessive sweating, sleeplessness, and headaches reported relief following gua-sha treatment.

In research conducted in 2014, gua-sha was proven to increase range of motion and lessen pain in people who frequently used computers. In addition, a 2017 study demonstrated that weightlifters who had gua-sha therapy were able to lift more weight.

Both gua-sha and a hot pack were effective in relieving the symptoms of elderly patients with back pain. The effects of gua-sha, on the other hand, lingered much longer. After a week, those who had gotten gua-sha treatment reported more mobility and reduced back discomfort than those who hadn't received treatment.

Effects Harmful to Health and Potential Hazards

Capillaries at the skin's surface are frequently ruptured by gua sha. "***Sha***" is the name given to the red or scarlet bruise that results. A few days to a few weeks is typical for the duration of the healing process.

Painkillers like Ibuprofen may be prescribed to alleviate discomfort and minimize bloating. The injured area should be protected, and care should be taken to avoid bumping it. Swelling and discomfort may be eased by applying a snowpack.

Risks exist, but Gua-sha specialists should not damage

your skin layer throughout the operation. Gua-sha practitioners should sanitize their instruments between treatments to prevent the spread of disease.

Gua-sha isn't for everyone, and those who should avoid it include the following:

- Those who have skin or vascular conditions that make stopping bleeding difficult.
- Those who are on blood-thinning medication or who have DVT are at an increased risk.
- Anyone who has had a wound that hasn't entirely healed, been contaminated, or has a tumor.
- A pacemaker or internal defibrillator is a good example of an implanted pacemaker.

Is Gua sha Painful?

Gua-sha intentionally inflicts bruising on its patients, which might cause some discomfort, but these bruises should recover within a few days.

Tools and Methods of the Gua-sha

Useful tools and equipment for Gua-Sha

In gua-sha, a curved-edged instrument is used. Scraping your skin with a spoon or coin is typically done, but in today's practice, therapists use a small hand-held tool with rounded edges to get the job done.

Tools used in gua-sha tend to be weighed to make applying pressure easier for the practitioner.

Practitioners of traditional East Asian medicine believe that certain stones, such as Bian rock, jade, and rose quartz, contain healing energies. IASTM and gua-sha in an infirmary frequently require medical-grade stainless steel. In order to get the most out of the equipment, professional therapists will use gas on the area of the body that is being treated.

The gua-sha practitioner will use smooth and strong strokes to insert these devices into the body. People may have to lie face down on a massage table if the Gua-sha technique is being used on the trunk or back from the legs outwards.

Chapter 6

Gua-Sha: The DIY Beauty Tool for an Inside-out Glow

When it comes to self-care and skin-care, ***Eva Ramirez*** examines the ancient ritual of Gua-sha and just how it could promote health insurance and radiance from the inside.

Traditional Chinese medicine's self-care technique known as gua-sha (***pronounced gwa-sha***) dates back thousands of years. Redirecting the flow of energy by scraping a tool over the skin is a way to reduce inflammation, increase blood flow, and stimulate lymphatic drainage, all of which help to promote healing in the human body. This simple but rigorous approach has been used for a very long time in the treatment of conditions like fever, muscle discomfort and pressure, swelling, recurrent coughs, sinusitis, and migraines. It is not for everyone.

Yang Sheng, the Chinese term for self-care, lies at the heart of Chinese medicine (healthy life). One of the many ancient wellness practices, Gua-sha, became increasingly popular in Western culture once it was used in the house. Many acupuncturists and therapists offer Gua-sha massage therapy, like cupping or acupressure, as an option. Similar to an athletic therapeutic massage but with a prop, it uses a medium to reduce pressure on a person's neck, legs, and arms, focusing on the specific areas that need attention. The bruising and inflammation caused by your frequent strokes can linger for a long time following treatment.

What are the Benefits of Dry Body Cleaning?

Do you think this has nothing to do with aesthetics or skin care? Well, a softer Gua-sha approach works like a miracle when applied to the skin on the face. You won't need to see a therapist in this situation because your routine daily skincare will take care of your skin's needs and well-being.

It's possible to heal Your Skin Layer with a Reiki Face.

A Gua-sha instrument and a minute-a-day application are

all that is required to see immediate effects and long-term advantages. It has also been shown to improve microcirculation by up to 100%, reduce wrinkles, rejuvenate and tone the skin, increase collagen, combat pigmentation, dark circles and puffiness under the eyes, define jawlines, and clear the sinuses.

It's literally like rubbing your path to healthy and glowing skin, because it primarily works from within and to the surface. You'll also notice a release of tension and a relaxing of facial muscles in the event that you clench your jaw at night. It's a practical way to alleviate any aches and pains you may be experiencing. There are many different ways to use the Gua-sha. You can use it to help, soothe, and calm muscles around your eyes if you get eye twitches because of insomnia or stress.

Jade gua-sha is the best way to ensure that you're utilizing the right tools for the job. Additionally, this green rock is respected because of its air-con capabilities and avoids anything made from bone or horn for obvious reasons. It's also a good idea to stay away from less expensive alternatives made from acrylic or other synthetic substances that could irritate your skin. The stone may glide more readily if you apply face oil to your skin before rubbing.

In the UK, Katie Brindle, a specialist in Chinese medicine, founded Hayo'u, an all-natural health insurance and skincare company. Simple daily routines and useful procedures make Chinese medicine's self-treatment component more accessible and approachable. The Gua-sha, which is normally carved from traditional Xiuyan jade and carries a velvet purse (great for traveling), as well as short, easy-to-follow films, are available for those who want to do the ritual at home.

Even if it's your first thing in the morning as a ritual or your last thing at night before turning in for the night, this calming and contemplative beauty routine can help you de-stress.

Chapter 7

How to Perform Gua-sha on a Face

Face Gua-Sha has a lot to offer

Eastern Botox refers to Gua-Sha, a treatment for facial and neck skin (or Eastern Facelift). When applied to the facial skin, this traditional Chinese medicine treatment accomplishes the following goals:

- Facial muscles that have begun to sag can benefit from this product.
- The top layer of skin is smoothed, and wrinkles on the face are reduced.
- Reduces the appearance of under-eye bags and dark circles (the type that comes with advancing age).
- Improves the appearance of wrinkles and other aging signs on the skin.
- In time, your skin tone becomes more rosy and vivacious.
- It can be used to treat skin conditions such as acne, rosacea, and other conditions of the epidermis on

the face.

Even though I've had positive encounters with Gua-Sha in the past, it's still a surprise to see how much my face has improved.

Face Gua-Sha has given me the clarity and luminosity that I'd only been able to get from taking Glutathione and Grape Seed pills before.

Detailed Step-by-step Instructions

As previously said, Gua-Sha is a centuries-old technique that calls for the use of a smooth-edged implement to scrape against the skin in circular motions all over the body. For the petechial, reddish stains that are the hallmark of Gua-Sha therapy, it is extremely difficult to raise them.

Gua-Sha Scraping

As your skin layer is scraped, the layers of your skin layer are activated and stagnant lymph that causes puffiness and a dull appearance is moved and cleared from the machine. Poisons will also be released, creating a brighter appearance, and finally, the massaging action relieves the anxious muscles that wrinkles provide.

Steps to Eastern Botox

Do not scrape the body with the same force with which you learned to scrape.you want this to function, only use light-weight materials. As a whole, the skin on the face is more sensitive.

The sluggish lymph is being flushed from your face by our therapists. We'll get rid of it by draining it through the appropriate lymphatic channels. Your collarbones are where you'll find these nooks and crannies.

Your entire scraping motion will be upwards only. Remember, we're trying to prevent sagging, so we can never do anything that might make things worse. If the dumping is performed in the lymphatic ducts described above, the only part that is excluded is the final product.

Cosmetic Gua-Sha

As a novice, here are the general steps you should take:

Third Vision: Your hairline or even closer to your eyebrows should feel like you've been hit by a heart attack. Curing is triggered in this area.

Lower forehead: Sweep from your stomach to your temples from the forehead over your eyebrows.

Under eyebrow: You can scrape the area underneath and above your eyelid with the curve of your gua-sha instrument. Be aware of the bone in the brow.

Under the eyebag: Beginning by gently stroking the medial side of your nasal bridge all the way up to your temple, your eye bags are most likely to appear. Consider pushing the sluggish lymph from your gills to your temples and all the way to your hairline as you do this.

Cheek: A similar sweeping motion can be used on the cheeks. Continue across your face or even further to the ear's inner lobe, depending on your preference.

Jaws: Sweep your lymphatic system up to your ears with the same motion you used for the jaws.

Chin: Sweep your chin from the center of your face to the lobes of your ears, making sure to go beneath your lower lip as well.

Under chin: Using your soft field under your chin, scrape from there to the base of your ear.

Throat: For the throat, a small amount of energy should be utilized to scrape the middle of the collarbone away from your mouth and earlobes.

Final step: As a final step, dump the lymph you've collected from the face into your lymphatic drainage. Then, using a circular motion, sweep your forehead, temples, and ears until you arrive at the throat and end of the lymphatic drainage. Repeat this process frequently to ensure thoroughness.

Chapter 8

How to Give Yourself the Best Facial Gua Sha at Home

What is the purpose of gua-sha?

When used to awaken meridians (*pathways of life energy*) and activate the body's inherent healing potential, gua-ha predates the more recent acupuncture technique. Collagen production *(power in cells)* is stimulated by gua sha, sculpting and shading the skin, allowing for the drainage of irritants as well as the relaxation of muscles, allowing them to establish their supporting channels effectively. Blood flow is usually increased, sending nutrition to areas that may have been starved due to blockage, which can help your skin get back to its most radiant condition.

As the meridian lines are enlivened, Gua-impact Sha's goes far beyond the skin's surface. The tummy, liver, spleen, heart, and kidneys all benefit greatly from this treatment, as does the rest of the body. Gua-sha tools can be used optimally if they are used over the area from the face to the kidneys.

What are the Huge Benefits?

- Provides your skin and tissues with a steady supply of nutrients and oxygen.
- purifies your cells by draining lymph fluid from your lymphatic system (which is typically full of toxins and waste).
- Reduces the appearance of wrinkles by at least half.
- Sagging of the skin is treated and prevented by using this product (which elevates and tightens your skin layer).
- Aids in the reduction of dark circles under the eyes.
- Assists in the removal of dark spots and hyperpigmentation from the skin.
- Improves the appearance of the skin.
- Increases the time it takes for outbreaks and acne to clear up. total assistance with these skin problems.
- Has the ability to treat and alleviate the symptoms of rosacea.
- Goodies to help with TMJ and migraines. product

penetration.

- It's an alternative to facelift surgery and injections (when used frequently in the home or when obtaining treatments from a qualified practitioner).

How will You Select a Gua-sha Tool?

Gua-sha tools come in a variety of shapes, sizes, and materials. Pet bone and horn are used in some devices, while jewels are used in others (like jade or increased quartz). Chinese soup spoons are used by a number of professionals. In a pinch, I've even seen the curved and soft-sided lid of a cup jar utilized.

Quartz and jade are the most popular gemstones at the moment.

Jade *creates an environment that is peaceful and pure, as well as fertile, harmonious, and restful.*

Rose quartz *is a powerful stone, establishing and aiding in the restoration of tranquility deep inside the heart, rose quartz. With its power to inspire compassion and unwavering care, it is known as the "Stone of Universal Love."*

The process of selecting a gua-sha rock resembles that of selecting a crystal or diamond. When you are able to pick it out yourself (please do that), Pick it up and hold it in your hands to get a feel for it. See which one catches your eye—if the first one shines brighter than the rest for you, go for it!

What's the Main Element to a Rewarding Practice?

Maintaining a healthy and blooming physique may require a regular regimen. Water, rest, healthy food, and physical activity are all part of our daily routine. Gua-sha therapy, on the other hand, is an investment that will pay off in the long run. The stomach is always the best choice because the body does not thrive when it is swinging between two extremes.

It's a good idea to incorporate this technique into your daily routine because your body uses 20 liters of fluid per day, and three liters of that fluid is lymph fluid. Gua-sha can be difficult to include in daily life, but carving out a few minutes a few days a week (even if it's just two minutes) is active. You may begin to recognize your body's desire for these self-care moments.

As you experiment with different levels of pressure, you'll need a light touch to ensure that you don't hurt yourself. The gua-sha rock should be swept across your face in a precise way. You're helping the lymph fluid more when you use a gentler touch, and increasing pressure indicates that you're working the muscles. Please take care not to inflict any harm on yourself or others.

How to Prepare Your Skin Layer

After cleansing your face, apply a hydrosol (I love True Botanicals Renew Nutrient Mist, OSEA's Sea Vitamin Boost, or Heritage Store's Rose Water), then apply facial oil (I love True Botanicals Renew Radiance Oil, OSEA's Undaria Argan Oil, or Shiva Rose Face Oil) around your face and neck using the fundamental oil left on your hands, and grease up your gua-sha tool with the remaining oil. Then get started, taking deep cleansing breaths while you do so.

How will You Perform Gua-sha?

Cleanse Face and Hands: After washing your hands and blow-drying your face with a clean washcloth, spritz your face liberally with a toner. With the hydrosol, you can get the essential oil, which you'll use next, deep into the epidermis and into the layers that need hydration and nourishment without having to use any additional products. When I finish using my washcloth, I put it in the hamper. If you suffer from acne, always wash your cosmetic towels before reusing them. Viruses and bacteria can be retransmitted through the skin.

Apply Facial: Start at the forehead and work your way down in the direction of the draining lymph liquid when applying Facial-Gas ***(from 4-10 drops).*** Before the gua-sha, this triggers movement in the epidermis and cells.

Rub the Gua-sha tool between your palms to warm it up a bit. You can slightly grease up the tool in this manner so that it doesn't draw on your skin in the areas that didn't receive much gas.

Sweep up your Adam's apple on both edges: Your REN collection may be activated instantly by gently swiping your Adam's apple on both sides; this is even more of an instant sweep. REN (the yin energy of the body) is collected by Chinese medicine through the REN channel, which guards against issues in the stomach area as well as the chest, neck, head, and face.

Sweep underneath your chin: Sweep beneath your chin, keeping your tool smooth as you go from your stomach to your earlobe. If you prefer, you can use your other thumb to support the skin beneath your chin while gliding these tools back to your earlobes in the opposite direction.

Sweep from the centre of the chin over your jawline: In order to stimulate the liquid to drain down the throat, you might gently wiggle your earlobes.

Sweep undern your cheekbone: Do not forget to sweep under your cheekbones. Grab a lot of liquid from this area and direct it toward your hairline. On the hairline, you can delicately wiggle your tool.

Sweep across your cheeks until you reach your hairline, then reapply.

My favorite way to focus my attention is by softly **swiping beneath my eye**. I love how my muscles and lymph flow down from my inner corner to my outer corner as I move my concentration toward my center of gravity. As an alternative, gua-sha can be done from the inside edge of a woman's care toward the hairline, which is the traditional method.

Sweep from the brow bone (in the forehead) all the way down to the hairline, finishing at the hairline: When sweeping down, work in small portions, traveling along the brow in three to five sections.

Sweep from the middle of your eyebrows over another eye or even more towards the hairline: Find out whether you're more psychic by swiping from the center of your eyebrows across another eye or even closer to the hairline.

Sweep through the centre from the forehead out to the hairline: Among the best treatments comes from Britta Plug of Britta Beauty in New York City, who sweeps from the forehead to the hairline. She doesn't touch the hairline as she moves into the locks, behind the ears, and down the throat from the forehead. I can't describe how good it feels.

Now caress the other part of your face: Once you've finished with your neck, move on to the other side of your face and repeat the process.

Sweep down your throat: Sweep down your throat once you've completed the other side of your face to help with long-lasting drainage. The tool should be positioned beneath your jawbone and gradually swept down your throat toward your collarbone while you keep it toned and steady.

Essential ideas to help you practice:

- I would recommend sweeping each area at least three times for extended practice, and up to ten times if possible.
- Rather than using the tool at a 90-degree angle to your skin layer, keep it at a 15-degree angle to it.
- Whenever you notice that your tool is pulling or drawing on your skin, administer a little more gas for a smoother ride.
- Try out different aspects and tools to see what works best for you. It's important to keep in mind that what's right for you may look different from what's shown in videos.

How often Should I Practice Gua-sha?

Gua-sha can be incorporated into a self-care routine every day, but if it begins to feel like an activity, take a break.

What does it Feel like?

Using admiring and gentle strokes with your touch is believed to be highly calming when done with gua-sha. You'll get the sensation of sweeping the gua-sha across the beautiful, delicate skin of a baby.

It's wonderful to be able to feel the fluids circulating. It's possible that you'll experience a reawakening of your skin's surface layer. Since the medial side of the feminine energy is said to be more employed when receiving, I frequently begin the medication on the left. When the rest of the body gets it, I've noticed that it primes the body's most responsive area.

How Excessive could Gua-sha be?

If you have recently had injections, avoid gua-sha. At the very least, **Botox** demands a two-week stay.

It's best to avoid using gua-sha on contaminated regions like cystic acne, pimples, and initial lesions, but it's a good idea to use gua-sha inside the breakout. Lymph can carry poisons toward the lymph nodes if it drains below the breakout.

Only perform each heart stroke ten times in the same area. If you keep repeating the sweep, you run the risk of activating the sensor too much. For example, it is possible to cause detoxification symptoms by moving an excessive amount of spleen at once with liquids (for example, dizziness or emotions of decrease with the flu).

Chapter 9

Cellulite

The gallbladder is the most common entry point for cellulite on the hips and thighs, as well as along the yang meridians. **Qi** in the gall bladder tends to be lower than in the other yang meridians because it is a smaller meridien. Subcutaneous fat protrudes into the dermis, forming an undulating junction between the epidermis and subcutaneous adipose cells and causing skin dimpling.

It is the spleen's job to distribute fat evenly throughout the body, particularly in the peripheral regions. When it comes to cellulite, your body's fat distribution is impaired, and some areas of your body appear to have no fat circulation at all. As a result of impaired circulation, there is little doubt that there is excess fat in the first place. As a result, we get the unbalanced visual we saw earlier.

In addition, we must address the meridian along which this problem occurs, which may be the gallbladder, the urinary bladder, or even the stomach, depending on the patient's condition. As a result, both the spleen and the corresponding meridian must be properly balanced.

Body Acupuncture Treatment

Cellulite on the outside of the thighs treated with acupuncture

- **Gall Bladder** - UB 19 (Back-Shu stage), GB 37 (Luo level).
- **Spleen** - UB 20 (Back-Shu period), St 40 (Luo place).
- Local needles and moving cup massage.
- There will be two sessions a week, totaling eight to ten sessions.

Atlanta divorce lawyers who are meridian-affected can use this therapeutic principle. The Bladder Meridian, for example, should be used in the Back-Shu posture (UB 28) and UB 58 (UB 28). (the Luo-connecting point of the yang meridian, to tonify the yang and reduce the yin aspect).

If done correctly, local therapy can be quite beneficial. Acupuncture cupping massage therapy isn't exactly enjoyable, so patients often desire to speed through the procedure.

Dedicated Local Treatment

If the problem area is along the gallbladder meridian, therapy should be performed in two halves, with the average person lying on one side and receiving all of the tiny needles and cupping first, before going through the other side and receiving the same treatment.

- Lying privately factors on your own body - UB 18, UB 20, St 40, GB 37.
- Approximately ten to fifteen local small needles of 0.20 mm gauge are inserted completely and perpendicularly at a distance of about three centimeters surrounding the cellulite at the same time.
- Both body needles and local needles are left in the body for 20 minutes.
- The cellulite should be treated with St. John's wort oil once all the needles have been removed. To avoid reducing friction in massage therapy, do not go overboard with this technique.
- For best results, use an open fire to create vacuum

pressure in a large cup (for a specific cellulite glass) and slide it along the area before the skin turns red. This is a painful method that can limit your vacuum's suction power if you're using it on a frequent basis. It only takes a few seconds to get a massage.

- After a treatment, the user may notice that his legs seem incredibly light.
- A course of treatment consists of eight to ten treatments given twice weekly.

What can an Average Person do at Home?

In order to avoid and increase circulation, which is the root cause of cellulite, the normal person can perform a slew of at-home remedies.

- Processed sweets, trans fats, and high-fat dairy products all contribute to weight gain by storing excess energy as fat in the body (though wholemeal, fruits, sugars, and honey are fine). These kinds of foods should be avoided at all costs.
- Blood flow is impeded when the fat tissue is

overly dense. As a result, it is critical that the ordinary person consistently consume clean water and stay hydrated throughout the day; consistency is more important than volume. Hot water surpasses cool, which is impressive and surmounts to how rapidly patients enjoy hot water, this is a remarkable achievement.

- A daily routine of rubbing and pummeling these areas with spiky toners will help break the stagnation of cellulite. For cellulite reduction, sitting cross-legged on the floor and moving sideways, forward, and backward for a quarter-hour a day in the privacy of your own house is a terrific option.

Gua-sha Massage for Cellulite Treatment

Do you have uneven, lumpy skin on your hips, thighs, or buttocks and want to get rid of it? Everything you need is in the Gua-sha Massage treatment for cellulite. You don't have to feel bad about how you look anymore. ***Meet Gua-Sha, the newest member of our family: Removing Cellulite.***

There are a variety of conditions that can benefit from the use of Gua-Sha massage therapy. These include lumbar stress, arthritis rheumatic, and heat stroke in the heart. The therapeutic effects of increased blood flow are triggered when the flow is activated, and this helps to alleviate blood stagnation.

Additionally, the Gua-sha Massage Cellulite helps to prevent new cellulite from forming.

Gua-Sha's benefits include: increased hydration, stress reduction, cellulite reduction, relaxation of facial muscles, increased blood flow, and more.

Treatment using Gua-sha Massage Therapy(GMT) includes:

There are many benefits to using a gentle scraping technique such as guasha to gently break up surface adhesions and stimulate circulation while also improving lymph drainage and firmness. As an added benefit, it reduces the appearance of fat cells and makes the skin appear smoother.

On any part of the body, you can perform gua-sha. It can be done on any area of the body, including the face, by an Atlanta divorce lawyer. It can help relax your skin's top layer, enhance facial blood flow, and boost collagen production, all of which improve the appearance of your skin's top layer and minimize the appearance of fine lines and wrinkles.

Cellulite removal may also be accomplished through the use of massage or dry brushing. An increase in blood flow and a reduction in the amount of discarded tissue can be achieved by stimulating cells manually. As a result, it enhances the skin's glow.

Free Bonus

Download "**The Magic Of Starting Over**" Ebook For **FREE!**

Did you know that the greatest barrier to success is the fear of failure? Fear of failure stops people from taking risks that might lead to success and triumph in overcoming obstacles.

Fear is part of human nature…

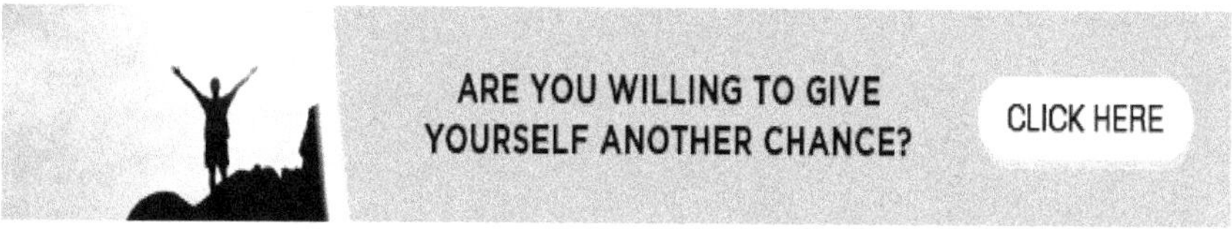

Click the image above to **Download the Book**, and also Subscribe for Free books, giveaways, and new releases by me. https://mayobook.com/marvin

Feedback

I'd like to express my gratitude to you for choosing to read this book, Thank you. I hope you got what you wanted from it. Your feedback as to whether I succeeded or not is greatly appreciated, as I went to great lengths to make it as helpful as possible.

I would be grateful if you could write me a review on the product detail page about how this book has helped you. Your review means a lot to me, as I would love to hear about your successes. Nothing makes me happier than knowing that my work has aided someone in achieving their goals and progressing in life; which would likewise motivate me to improve and serve you better, and also encourage other readers to get influenced positively by my work. Your feedback means so much to me, and I will never take it for granted.

However, if there is something you would love to tell me as to improve on my work, it is possible that you are not impressed enough, or you have a suggestion, errors, recommendation, or criticism for us to improve on; we are profoundly sorry for your experience (remember, we are human, we are not perfect, and we are constantly striving to improve).

Rather than leaving your displeasure feedback on the retail product page of this book, please send your feedback, suggestion, or complaint to us via E-mail to **"marvin@mayobook.com"** so that action can be taken quickly to ensure necessary correction, improvement, and implementation for the better reading experience.

I'm honored that you've read this book and that you enjoy it. I strive to provide you with the best reading experience possible.

Thank you, have a wonderful day!

About The Author

Marvin Valerie Georgia is the founder and CEO of Healthy-Lifestyle-Movement, a coaching company that specializes in general medicine, human psychology, parenting, and stress management. Her goal is to help people live their healthiest and happiest lives possible.

Marvin Valerie has been in the business of coaching and consulting since 2005. As a professional, she has experience with a variety of health conditions such as hypertension, diabetes, cardiovascular disease, high cholesterol, and osteoporosis. She believes that when it comes to good health, it's all about balance. In her personal life, she strives to maintain a healthy lifestyle by eating well, exercising, and keeping stress at bay.

Marvin and Valerie's goal is to help people live their healthiest and happiest lives possible. To accomplish this goal, she uses a holistic approach that includes nutrition, exercise, psychology, and stress management. She believes that good health starts from the inside out and is the foundation for living a happy life.

Subscribe to my Newsletter to download my Free Book,

and also be informed about my new releases, and giveaways here: https://mayobook.com/marvin

Connect with me on my Facebook Page here: https://fb.me/Marvinvaleriegeorgia

My Other Books

I recommend these books to you, they will be of help, check them out after reading this book.

1. **Acupuncture:** A Practical Guide to Enjoying a Perfect Health with Natural Medicine
2. **Alcohol Control:** The Guide to Overcoming Alcoholism, and Breaking Free From Alcohol Addiction (Alcoholism Recovery)
3. **Alcohol Detox:** The Guide to Safely Clean Up Your Lifestyle, Detoxify & Maintain Healthy Body Without Drugs (Alcoholism Recovery)
4. **Anger Management:** The Inside Out Parent Child Interaction Therapy (PCIT) Approach to Managing Anger Issues and Emotions (Anger Management Program Book 1)
5. **CBT - Cognitive Behavioral Therapy:** The Clinician & Parental Guide to Managing Anger, Anxiety, ADHD, Trauma, Conduct Disorder, and Overcoming Negative
6. **ADHD:** A Practical Parental & Educator Multimodal Guide to Helping Children with ADHD Break Through Barriers and Develop Ability to Regulate their Behaviors and Strengths
7. **Asthma Relief:** How To Relieve Your Asthma Symptoms And Live The Life You Deserve with Natural Remedies
8. **7-Day Cleanse and Detox:** The Ultimate Guide To Getting Clean And Feeling Good!
9. **Cognitive Behavioral Therapy for Conduct Disorders**

and Personality Disorders: How to Use CBT to Help Kids with Emotional Disorders

10. **Dyslexia:** Things You Don't Know About Dyslexia Learning Difficulties (But Should)
11. **Fear:** Overcoming and Facing Your Fear & Succeeding at Anything
12. **Sensory Processing Disorder:** How to Help Kids Cope with Sensory Issues (SPD)
13. **How to Parent - Toddler Discipline:** Raising Happy, Well-Behaved Kids by Taming the Tantrum Monster
14. **Childhood Trauma Healing:** Understanding & Healing Traumatic Experiences that Affect Children's Wellbeing (Emotional Trauma and Recovery Guide)
15. **Gua Sha:** An Ancient Chinese Technique for Facial and Skin Self Healing
16. **Potty Chair for Boys and Girls:** Potty Training in One Week, and The Ultimate Potty Buying Guide
17. **ADHD in Kids: ADHD in Kids:** What Parents and Teachers Should Know About Attention Deficit Hyperactivity Disorder

CPSIA information can be obtained
at www.ICGtesting.com
Printed in the USA
LVHW080103080922
727808LV00004B/759

9 781637 503331